#1 In a Series

Murder by Medicine Is No Accident...

THE LETHAL DOSE

WHY YOUR DOCTOR IS PRESCRIBING IT

By Dr. Jennifer Daniels, MD, MBA

Copyright 2013 by Dr. Jennifer Daniels, MD, MBA.

All rights reserved.

No part of this book may be reproduced in any form or by any electronic means or mechanical means, including information storage and retrieval systems, without permission in writing from the publisher, expect by a reviewer or where copyright law allows.

DISCLAIMER

This document is a combination of information found in medical literature and information acquired through clinical observation by Dr. Jennifer Daniels in her medical clinical practice. It should not be construed as medical advice. You are advised to consult with your physician in regards to any medical decision that may relate to your health. This information is for informational purposes only. Nothing, including communications with Dr. Daniels, should be taken as medical advice. You should not act upon anything without first discussing it with your physician. The information in this document is designed for educational purposes only, so that you might better understand your condition. Any information is provided as is, with all faults, with no representations or warranties of any kind expressed or implied, including but not limited to implied warranties of merchantability or fitness for a particular purpose. You assume total responsibility and risk for using this information and any sources related to it. No oral or written information shall take precedence over this warranty. In no event will Everyday Vitality LLC, its employees, directors, or agents be liable to you or anyone else for any decision made or action taken in reliance upon the information provided herein.

INTRODUCTION

This book is a brief overview of Dr. Daniels experiences, observations and conclusions about medicine during her 34 years of being in the Medical profession.

Dr. Jennifer Daniels trained as a medical doctor and received a medical degree from the University of Pennsylvania School of medicine and an MBA in health care administration from the Wharton School. Her premedical studies were completed at Harvard University. For 10 years, Dr. Daniels practiced as a board-certified family practice physician. At that point, the farthest thing from her mind was the idea that the health care she was trained to deliver might actually be lethal. As this awareness crept up on her, she noticed that properly treated and fully compliant patients appeared to be getting sicker. It became apparent to Dr. Daniels that it was not a healthcare system, not a disease curing system, at all. In fact, this health care system is a disease creation system that she was enmeshed in. This is her story, and how she is working to reverse the tide.

DEDICATION

This book is dedicated to all those whose lives were cut short by medicine and to those who will live a longer, happier lives as a result of the information in this book. This book is also dedicated to my children who adjusted to growing up different than most Americans, to my mother who let me see the world through a different set of lenses, and the thousands of patients who contributed to my re-education.

TABLE OF CONTENTS

THE LETHAL DOSE 1

THE NUMBERS POINT TO HOMICIDE 9

THE AWAKENING 13

NO CURES ALLOWED 19

GETTING BETTER VS. GETTING WORSE 25

PAYING THE PRICE FOR HELPING THE COMMUNITY 34

MAKING MONEY IN THE HOSPITAL, DEAD OR ALIVE ... 40

PRESCRIPTION DRUGS 46

DRUG TOXICITY AND THE TRUTH ABOUT THE
PHARMCUTICAL DRUG MODEL 52

DOCTORS ARE HOLOGRAMS 60

WRITING RECIPES ON MY PRESCRIPTION PAD 66

MORE ABOUT NATURAL REMEDIES 73

HOW TO POOP: VITALITY PURGING CAPSULES 76

CONTINUING LEARNING MORE ABOUT NATURAL
REMEDIES 80

RESOURCES 83

ENDNOTES 84

Dr. Jennifer Daniels

THE LETHAL DOSE

Adequately discussing the lethal dose and why your doctor is most certainly prescribing it demands that I first define lethal and how that concept was introduced to me in medical school. Lethal dose is the amount of something, usually a medication or a chemical, that causes death. In medical school, we were taught about something called LD50. LD 50 is the dose of a drug which 50% of those who take it die, actually drop dead. This is a pretty high bar to pass. In other words, something that killed 15% of those who take it would not be considered a lethal dose. You can imagine to my young tender 22-year-old ears that the thought of administering anything that could kill half of the people who receive it was just appalling and shocking. So of course, I asked the unthinkable question: "What about the LD0?" What about giving the dose of the medication that didn't kill anybody? When I asked this question, I was told there was no such dose. Somebody's going to die at every dose, but the benefits outweigh the risk. Further, the importance of medical training was to teach the elite (that was me) how to safely recommend drugs that were so powerful they could cure or kill. This is why it is so important to stick to protocols and the Standard of Care.

The thought that I was being trained to recommend deadly therapies troubled me. What benefit to the patient was more important than life itself? How could being killed by a medicine be better than living with an illness? I could tell I had a lot to learn. The professors' answers to prior questions ran through my mind: research is ongoing; better solutions would be found; the benefits of therapy outweigh the risk of death; and even though things might not be as safe as we like right now, they're getting safer every day. So that's how the concept of the lethal dose was introduced in medical school.

One day, it finally occurred to me: there are no benefits. Coumadin is the drug that impressed this on my consciousness. You may know someone who takes it, or you may have heard of it. It helps thin the blood, and there's this condition called atrial fibrillation where the heartbeat is irregular. In Medical School we were taught that when a person first gets an irregular heartbeat, it's very important to thin their blood for a period of three months with this special medicine and then stop the medicine because it saves lives. I said to the professor: "Wait a minute, if this drug is so good, why don't we continue it longer? Why don't we do even more good?"

He said, "Well, the reason we don't continue it more than three months is because at the three month point, the number of lives saved by preventing a stroke due to atrial fibrillation is equal to the number of deaths caused by the drug when people bleed to death from it. After the three months of taking the drug, the deaths from Coumadin exceed deaths resulting from untreated Atrial Fibrillation. So, at the three month point then, everything's a wash. I found this a little troubling because I was being trained to give a drug to kill as many people as it would have saved. The goal of saving lives is not accomplished. So the total number of people who died is the same whether I give the drug or whether I don't because the dose of this drug that I'm giving is guaranteed to create at least as many deaths as lives it saves. Now another odd thing about this is the obvious conflict of interest: allowing the manufacturers of the drug to decide how many lives the drug is really saving and how many lives the drug is really taking in terms of murdering people. Clearly, if someone is making this drug they're going to overestimate the number of deaths the drug prevents and underestimate the number of deaths the drug causes. There's plenty of evidence that this is exactly what has happened. The evidence is literally 107,000 people every single year who die for properly prescribed medication.

These are highly trained doctors who have done their reading and who have kept up with research, and yet they are literally prescribing lethal doses of medication. It might not shock you, but that's actually more than the deaths caused by incompetent doctors. That's right. Your chances of being a victim of medical homicide are actually greater the more highly trained your doctor is and the more competent your doctor is. So the troubling thing of course is the underestimation of the deaths created by the drug, overestimation of the benefit of the drug, and who is making this decision on these numbers. So, it turns out that the lethal dose of medication is equal to the therapeutic dose. And so, just by following the Standard of Care, a doctor does a lot of harm. Now there are drugs that have been identified as especially dangerous and whenever this happens, the FDA puts down their foot. What happens then is the FDA demands that the drug company, through the FDA, do a special mailing to doctors and mail them a special notice telling them this drug is really dangerous; it's killed a lot of people, and we want you take the following precautions.

I will give you the example of this. Doctors, by the way, get this mail frequently. This one drug I want to mention is something called Brilinta. And not that Brilinta is especially bad. It is very typical. I want to show you some examples so we can point out the things that happen when doctors are educated. These are things that lead them to actually prescribe a drug in its deadly dose even more often as a result of the training. So Brilinta is a drug that is prescribed to help thin the blood and this is believed to prevent heart attacks. Now it's important to know that if you have a heart attack, the time where you get chest pain, you clutch your chest, then your chances of dying of a heart attack are 3.6%. In other words, if a cat has 9 lives, then the average human has 24 heart attacks before they actually die. This is an important thing to understand as you assess the relative benefits of this drug. So Brilinta has a gross death rate of 2.6% per year of use. The death rate from heart disease is 35% in a lifetime. The risk of a person dying of a heart attack is less than one percent in any given year. So you're going to take a blood thinning medication that gives you 2.6% per year death rate in order to avoid a heart attack which has at most a 1% death rate. So we already have a drug that's more than twice as deadly as the disease it's supposed to prevent. Now that would be okay if that's all it was, but it turns out, with this drug you have an 11% chance of bleeding so severely that you require more than four units of blood to be transfused. This is the special alert that they sent to doctors. So they explained it to the doctors, and then told the doctors to don't ever stop this drug. The only time you can stop this drug is if you contact the doctor who originally prescribed the drug. Nowadays with medical care, you have group practices. As such, a doctor might change from one group to another group, might move to another state, might not be on call, and so you're only allowed to stop this drug once you talk to the prescribing doctor. So you have a patient who's bleeding to death, and you're transfusing blood. You're on your 4th unit, the 6th unit, you pump it into him and you should never stop this drug that caused the bleeding until you talk to the doctor who prescribed it. Now you would think that in the literature they mail to the doctor they would say, now when you call the doctor who initiated the drug, this is what that doctor will do... There is no mention anywhere in the literature mailed to the doctor as to what the doctor will do once he is contacted. There literally is no provision for this drug to ever be stopped even as it's causing the patient to die. So this is actually shocking. Had a doctor not receive this notice in the mail he might have said look, the medicine causes bleeding. If she gets a little bleeding, I'll just stop the drug. Yet this written instruction to the doctor is very clear. No, you are not to stop the drug. Now a sensible thinking individual would say, "That's ridicu-

The Lethal Dose

lous. I'm a doctor, and I can decide to stop the drug and absolutely not kill somebody with the drug. And it turns out that your doctor knows what to prescribe because he follows something called the Standard of Care. And within the Standard of Care is these written instructions the doctor receives from the drug company and from the FDA. So doctor receives this instruction, this is the Standard of Care.

The Standard of Care is transmitted to doctors through these mailings, through continuing medical education conferences, and textbooks. It's not something he's free to ignore. When doctors ignore the Standard of Care, they can lose their hospital privileges, and therefore their right to earn money by working at hospitals. They can be subject to malpractice lawsuits because malpractice law is very clear and says that if a doctor fails to adhere to the Standard of Care, then he can be found libel. So the doctor's in a little bit of a pickle here. If he refuses to prescribe the lethal dose, then he can actually be prosecuted in court for failure to adhere to the Standard of Care. Now, you can imagine this is a high stress situation to be in. Another situation with the Standard of Care is insurance payment. Insurance companies inform the doctors that if the doctor does not adhere to the Standard of Care, then the insurance company will refuse to compensate or pay the doctor for his services. Also, the Standard of Care is linked to licensure. And in licensure, if the doctor failed to adhere to the Standard of Care, he can be investigated by a licensing board and have his license removed; in this case literally for failure to commit medical homicide. And so that's a lot of pressure on him to literally prescribe the lethal dose.

And so to ask the question, where does the Standard of Care really come from? Who writes this? Who has this authority? It turns out there are only three entities that can write the Standard of Care. One is the drug company. The drug companies develop the drug, and they write the Standard of Care they believe to be the proper use of this drug. And of course they write this to maximize their revenue and the economic impact of the drug. This is given special importance once it receives FDA approval prior to marketing. Insurance companies can also write the Standard of Care; they can write it into contracts that Doctors sign. When Insurance companies write the Standard of Care, they seek to maximize their particular profits. And of course, hospitals can also write the Standard of Care, and they write the Standard of Care, again, to ensure their economic viability, another term for profits. Who cannot write the Standard of Care? Doctors cannot write the Standard of Care. So as a doctor in a private office, I cannot say, "Wait a minute, I've seen three patients die already. I followed the Standard of Care, and they have done very poorly. They died. So I'm going to write a new Standard of Care where I will no longer prescribe or administer this particular medication." Doctors do not have that authority. And guess who else is not allowed to write the Standard of Care? Patients are not permitted to write the Standard of Care.

The Lethal Dose

This became a huge political issue. Many years ago patients with Lyme disease determined that they needed a longer course of antibiotics in order to get relief from their illness. Most doctors refused to prescribe the longer courses of antibiotics, and the doctors that did were prosecuted and lost their licenses. Through a lot of litigation, political activity, and funding their own research, they were able to get this one little Standard of Care altered. Still, this very wealthy and educated group of people found that patients are not permitted to initiate or alter the Standard of Care.

So we have system where a doctor is obligated to follow treatment protocols that are apparently lethal and inherently biased, much to the detriment of his patient. So this is why it's likely that your doctor is prescribing the lethal dose. It's really important that people understand these facts because so many people say. "No, I know a lot of people dying from medical care, but it couldn't happen to me. It couldn't happen to me because my doctor's well trained, my doctor's competent, and he's prescribing drugs according to the Standard of Care." That is exactly how death by medicine occurs, and that actually puts you at very high risk of death.

Dr. Jennifer Daniels

THE NUMBERS POINT TO HOMICIDE

Let do a little rundown of some causes of death by medicine. These examples are not disputed by anyone. It is well agreed upon by the government and medical authorities that these deaths occur.

Condition	Deaths	Reference
Hospital ADR/med error	420,000	Leape[1], NPSF[2]
Nursing Home / Malnutrition	4,630	Coalition for Nursing Home Reform[3]
Outpatients	199,000	Null, Gary (2011-10-16)[4]
Unnecessary Procedures	37,136	Death by Medicine (Kindle Locations 327-357)[4]
Surgery Related	32,000	NBN_Mobi_Kindle[4]
Hospital Acquired Infections	99,000	"Hospital-acquired infections FAQ."[5]
Bedsores from Hospital	60,000	AHRQ[6]
Total	851,766	

The Lethal Dose

As much as 107,000 people die every year from properly prescribed medications. This means that doctors doing the right thing and just following orders leads to death. This figure is confirmed by the journal of American Medical Association. Then the figure is 92,000 deaths every year by doctors who are incompetent, doctors who deviate from the Standard of Care. This is confirmed by the National Safety Council. These are the same folks who count car accidents and other such things. These are subsumed in the 420,00 figure above. Next, there's a figure of 99,000 deaths every year from hospital acquired infection. This is confirmed by the Extended Cure Study and several other studies that put the number at or around 99,000. (There are studies that put this number much higher than that, but I'm going to give them the benefit of the doubt just to be safe). There are 60,000 people every year that die because they go into facilities and they get bedsores.

Now the grand total here is 851,766 people a year. This is admittedly a very low figure because it only counts deaths acknowledged by the health care industry.

Because this number is so huge, I'd like to try and put it in perspective for you. The United States has been engaged in a war with Iraq. Now with all of our drone missiles, our fighter jets, artillery, all the arsenal, all the equipment and implements of war, the only thing that's been able to happen is we've only got a death number of 233,000 over the 40 month period of March 2003 to June 2006. I pick this period because it is the one for which a credible source, the New England Journal of Medicine[7], provides information. So if you divide 233,000 by 40 and multiply by 12 the annual kill comes to 69,900 casualties per year. There are 33 million Iraqis. With 69,900 deaths a year per 33 million, this is a .21% kill rate per year. The U.S. Military in Iraq, using the latest in technology, kills .21% of the population each year.

There are 313 million United States citizens, and the health care system is murdering at least 851,766 each year; this equates to a .27% kill rate per year in the United States. This is a kill rate that is 0.27 / 0.21% or 129% the kill rate our military has in a country where we are at war and actually making a deliberate, well planned effort to harm the people in that country. This has led me to conclude two things. One, we need to replace our military with our health care system, and it would be more efficient than our military in exterminating our enemies. Using the health care may result in 129 percent of the Iraqi fatalities and there would be no US casualties. In other words, we should simply invite our enemies to partake of our healthcare system free of charge and then the kill rate would increase to 129% of the present kill rate with only Iraqi casualties. Far more efficient than what's being experienced with all of our military. The second conclusion this comparison suggests is that the health care system in the United States is a deliberate, coordinated effort to murder Americans. Is this really homicide? You bet it is. When you think of it, there is no other way to look at this except that it is homicide. I'd like to make people more aware of this and to help them determine what their risk is. This is the leading cause of death in the United Stated

The Lethal Dose

and people are dying all the time because they don't really feel they're at risk.

Iraqis know that they are at war and I'll bet you that when they see an armed American soldier, they do not run to him and ask him for an appointment. They don't pay for parking, and stand in line to get murdered. In fact I'll bet you dollars to donuts they probably run the other way. They'll run and hide. They might even stay very quiet hoping that the soldier will walk by their house and not realize that they're there. Another thing that they don't do is they don't take out a special insurance policy to make sure that their executioners get paid a little extra once they die. So what the Iraqis have done is they have taken evasive action. They have tried to make really sure that the people who've arrived in their soil to execute them do not receive any reward for doing so. So it might be that a similar posture is called for the part of patients and everyday citizens in the United States with respect to the health care system.

Dr. Jennifer Daniels

THE AWAKENING

My name is Dr. Jennifer Daniels. I'm trained in allopathic medicine, graduated from Harvard in 1979, and graduated University of Pennsylvania School of Medicine and Wharton School in 1983. I stayed in medical practice for 10 years, and saw that my patients weren't getting well. After taking a deeper look into the whole field of prescription medication, I ended up changing my medical practice.

I sensed that something was wrong about our medical system as early as high school. I was a candy striper (volunteer) at the local teaching hospital. One of my many responsibilities was to escort patients from their car to admissions and from their hospital room to their car on discharge. Without fail, people were optimistic, cheerful on admission and whimpering, wrapped in bandages, and filled with suffering and pain on discharge. My concern deepened as an undergraduate at Harvard. At Harvard, my grades were excellent. So, it looked like things were going well; and getting into medical school was a 100 percent sure shot. Now as much as then, my goal is to uplift humanity by improving the health of individuals so they would live longer, better lives, be happier, and have an opportunity for all the great things that life is supposed to be filled with!

The Lethal Dose

So I decided to go to the Weidner Library to check this out and get my plan together. I really wanted to be an effective member of the medical field. Weidner Library is a world-famous library located within the Harvard campus. Anything you wanted was in that library. If it wasn't, they could get it for you. I even had access to the congressional record! That was impressive since this was before everyone had the internet readily available to them.

So I checked out a ton of books and started reading them, and then my heart just sank. And I read that *access to medical care and receiving medical care had zero, zippo input or benefit to the health of a population*. Naturally, I was confused. What was it I was working for then? What was the medical field and technology really accomplishing?

So after all this money, time, and hard work—Harvard wasn't easy or particularly fun—they are telling me in several different books that medicine and medical care is not what made people healthy. Let me say that again: *health care does not make people healthy and does not improve their outcome or their life.*

A panic set in. At this point, I began to worry about things like, "How am I going to get paid? How can I make sure my patients benefit?" I thought I'd go to Harvard, become a doctor, and everything would be fine. So then I started reading congressional reports, because as early as 1977, Kennedy proposed a national health insurance plan. Then I started reading and reading and reading it, and I was like, "Wait a minute! This health care plan is not making any sense! *It's just a blank check to anyone in the health care field. There's nothing in this bill about anyone benefitting or even receiving health care for that matter*!" It was all about submitting bills and getting money.

I decided to continue medical school since I was already so far into it and there was promising research that might improve the effectiveness of medicine. However, I couldn't bring myself to borrow even a single penny to pay for my education. I figured that if what I'm doing is not really valuable, then people probably won't be paying me for it anyway. I would learn everything I could, and hope that maybe I'd get something useful out of it all. From there, I knew I could continue to educate myself, and eventually I assumed that I would find a way to bring value and usefulness to my chosen field. I'd find a way to help people get healthy."

That was my naïve, 22-year-old view of the world. Luckily Harvard wasn't nearly as expensive back then. At around $8,000 per year, it was a mere pittance compared to costs now. Back in 1979, that was a lot of money, but nothing like tuition costs today. $8,000 was about half of an average person's annual income in the United States. Now, the price of Harvard is more than the median income at more than $50,000 year. Proportionally the cost has exploded, but back then it was manageable. To pay for Harvard, I sold books door to door 14 hours a day during summer vacations.

The Lethal Dose

Of course, I got into medical school. I was admitted by 13 different medical schools, so I had my pick. I settled on University of Pennsylvania because there's a business school across the street (The Wharton School), and I could get both degrees during the same four years.

At medical school, I had the same types of revelations, only it wasn't text books anymore. It was practical and tangible, and I kept saying to myself, "Wait a minute. *I don't see anybody getting better here.* Where are the success stories? Where are the healing stories? What's going on here?" I returned to the library to find out more about the ineffectiveness of medicine. There were no books on the subject in the libraries I had access to.

So I started asking my professors, but that didn't seem to help me with my conundrum much. I even went to the dean, and I said to him, "I came from the ghettos of Syracuse, and I can't take this stuff back to the ghetto. Man, they are going to eat me alive. They don't believe in malpractice; they believe in *getting even!* Tell *me* something. This is not going to work!"

I was sincere and earnestly concerned. But here is this white-haired, white guy—I mean, how could he even stifle a giggle! I explained the situation I was returning to after Medical school, and told him that I really needed some *useful information.*

He said, "Well, Jennifer, calm down, calm down. We're getting to the good part. You're going to learn the cures next semester. Next semester we'll tell you the good stuff." So I took a deep breath and took him at his word.

The next semester, I took medical school extremely seriously. I woke up early every day, and I studied extremely late every night. I even ate every other day because if you eat every day then you sacrifice the amount of time it takes to eat. Think about it: it takes time to get to the restaurant; it takes time to get served; it takes time to eat; and it takes time to get back to the library. It's a whole hour or two per meal, right? So I calculated that if I eat every other day, I would have that much more time to study. I was really intense about this.

And so of course, as you might imagine, *at the end of the semester, there were no success stories*. And so each semester I kept going back to the dean and saying, "Hey, hey, hey, when's it coming, when's it coming?"

So finally graduation shows up. And I said, "Well, wait a minute. I still don't have anything I can take back to the ghetto. At least nothing I can take back and not be abused for my lack of effectiveness."

So the dean says, "Don't worry, Dr. Daniels. Just continue your medical education. There's also a residency, and pay close attention to your residency. *You'll learn a lot in your residency*, and keep up with Continuing Medical Education (CME) seminars. That is the place where the best therapies are revealed first"

Are you starting to see a pattern?

Dr. Jennifer Daniels

NO CURES ALLOWED

I went on with my residency, but it was practically mass murder. The only thing that kept me going was the manner in which they sleep-deprived us. They work you for more than 90 hours a week, so there's not a lot of time for reflection. There wasn't a bunch of time to say, *"Hey, what if the District Attorney busted this joint, where would I be?"* You simply don't have time for that thought processes. So as a resident, I just kept slugging it out every day; just doing the best that I could. You're trying to help as many patients as you can, and it wears you down. From there, at *every point your best interests are pitted against the best interest of the patient.* Let me tell you a couple of stories.

As students, we certainly weren't allowed to have any bright ideas. W*e were not allowed to offer any solution or thought that was outside of something that would profit the drug company or hospitals.* One might assume that the paradigm that was taught would be that these drugs are helping to cure disease. That isn't the case at all. In fact, that *was never said.* The administration was extremely stern on this fact. As a resident, you were never allowed to use the *"Cure"* word. No matter what, we could never tell the patient we were curing them. So I had natural questions like, "What are we here for then?"

The Lethal Dose

My intention going into the medical field was to help cure people, help those live betters, longer lives. Yet they said, "You cannot use that word. We are not curing *anything*. We are *treating* the patient. This is *treatment*. We want to be sure to give the patient *proper treatment*." I'd spent so much of my life studying this, and invested so much time and so much money and had so much confidence in how true this cause is and how helpful I could be toward other people. I wanted to tell the patients, "I can help you. I can *cure* you." But the senior doctor says, "Whoa, whoa, whoa, back up, back up; you can't *do* that."

As a medical student you are doing the scut work that no one else wants to do. So one time, it was my job to do a complete physical exam and to ask the patient questions before surgery. This patient came in for surgery on his trigger finger, and it was bent. Actually it wasn't a trigger; it was a frozen finger, a frozen joint, and it was bent. He couldn't do much with this finger. I ended up asking the "wrong" question. This was a question that literally cost the hospital over $5,000. So as you might imagine, I was not popular.

So I examined this person, examined the finger, examined the hand, documented everything, and I said to the patient, "Mr. Jones, what are you *expecting* as a result of this surgery? *Exactly what outcome are you expecting*?"

He said, "Well, see this finger? I want to be able to straighten this finger and to bend it and to straighten it and to have full control of that finger." I documented that in the chart that full use is exactly what he wanted and even expected.

Well, medicine can't give that. All they can do is freeze the finger in a different position, and that's what they had planned for him. But *he didn't know that*. So they were going to take this guy to surgery, charge thousands of dollars for OR time; the hand specialist was going to make thousands of dollars, the hospital was going to get thousands of dollars for the bed space and all this other stuff; and a lot more money spent in rehab. This whole $5,000 to $10,000 experience was planned. However, when they read my chart, my note, and this patient's expectation before surgery, *they had to cancel everything. They could not defraud this guy; they could not strip him of his wealth and mutilate his body because some little medical student asked the wrong question.*

They didn't tell him that this procedure was going to make his trigger finger nice and straight, but they allowed him to believe what he wanted about the whole process. They never considered asking him about his expectations. Sadly, *that is the whole story of medicine*. This is just a little, itty bitty snapshot, but that is the story of *every single medical encounter*!

The person needing medical attention is <u>presold</u>. These are all marketing terms: "presold" by the media. *The same lies they taught me in medical school, they are teaching kids in health class as early as first grade.* So they are getting these kids presold and prepared to believe in the concept of "medical benefit without cure."

And "medical benefit" is a term like 'orange.' So "medical benefit" doesn't mean the patient benefits. *"Medical benefit" is something the doctors do*, called a "benefit." Society programs children and young adults this way, and so they are ready to submit to this idea of medical benefit. It's like saying, "Oh, yep, I had this surgery and it didn't benefit me–no, I'm not any better off after the surgery, but I do have a medical benefit because I came out of the hospital alive."

So we either submit to this or start asking ourselves, "What exactly is a 'benefit' anyway?"

Of course, I thought I did a good job: I did a complete physical, and I asked all the questions. I documented everything. The next day, I was not on the good guy list. They were livid. I was a little concerned that maybe I had just damaged my medical school career. I began to worry about how bad of a mistake I'd made and if I'd actually end up graduating. I nearly lost my license before I even got it good.

Let me digress a little bit and talk about continuing my education after medical school. I subscribed to the cassette tapes available back then. These ranged from topics on pediatrics, obstetrics and gynecology, family practice, internal medicine, etc. I was getting a blizzard of these tapes every month, listening to every last one of them, to make sure I heard every word. Then I'd listen again. After my medical education, I would have spent my whole frigging paycheck if that's what it took to make sure I did not miss a single medical breakthrough. Those long driving distances in Wisconsin came in handy.

I was horrified. I was horrified because here I was working as a family practice physician. I spent a lot of time treating hypertension, for example. I was pressuring myself to get this right. It was my job to get that blood pressure down, give patients that water pill. Then the water pill lowers their potassium (this could kill the patient), so I had to give them potassium and try to keep all of these details balanced. I had to work hard so I didn't kill anybody.

I was horrified because I received a cassette in the mail that tells me, *"The treatment of hypertension does not increase life expectancy by one day."*

This is worse than the story I heard back in medical school. They told me weren't curing people. I did not realize we were not even improving their health. I still couldn't understand it. Are these people seriously telling me that as a medical professional, I am obligated to provide ineffective therapy? *So here I was spending my day treating high blood pressure / hypertension with medications that do not extend lifetime.* (This is still the standard treatment by the way). So I said, "Well, why am I doing this? Why are we still doing this?" I even took this question to the podium at one of the CME conferences.

The Lethal Dose

Every authority on the matter told me the same thing. *"You are doing this because this is the best therapy we have available, and research is going to produce breakthroughs that will have more effective therapy in the future, but until then we are doctors and we are obligated to do what we have set out in front of us."*

The recurring theme: no cures allowed. Period.

Dr. Jennifer Daniels

GETTING BETTER VS. GETTING WORSE

After my stint at Harvard, I went on to University of Pennsylvania School of Medicine. Not only would I continue my medical education, but I'd attend Wharton School for an MBA in Business as well. I planned to go back to the ghetto, and needed an answer to the questions: "How do you get blood out of a stone? How am I going to collect enough money to keep my medical office open in this drug and crime-ridden ghetto?"

I went to business school to help me figure out how to face this challenge. This was during the same time I only ate every other day, and I spent almost all of my time focused on my studies in medicine and business. Naturally, I was pretty skinny at the time. Being on an every-other-day fast, was not only healthy for me in certain ways, but it also helped me afford to continue school and reach all of my goals.

After graduating at Wharton and Pennsylvania School of Medicine, my original plans to return home and work with those in need throughout the ghetto was put on hold. I took a minor detour. It was 1983, and having decided to completely avoid loans to pay for school — because the information they were teaching me wasn't

The Lethal Dose

worth ten cents—I didn't have any debt. But, I had signed up for the National Health Service Corps when I entered medical school. Under this program, I agreed to work in an underserved area for each year that the government paid for me to go to medical school.

I kept my promise to the National Health Service Corps. I headed out West. I went to Wisconsin for 18 months then North Dakota. I worked as the medical director. The Corps were extremely happy that I had an MBA, and had administrative skills needed to upgrade the clinics. The clinic I worked at was located on the Indian reservation. That was a real eye-opener *because we had been told in medical school that the reason our patients weren't getting better is because they were poor, and they were ignorant, and they weren't following our instructions.*

Basically, we were taught to blame the patient. We were taught to blame the patient every single time. And so then I said, "Okay, here I am on the Indian reservation." I am in charge. I can solve this problem. There will be compliance. We had special funding. It was a self-determined tribe, which means they could hire me because they felt like it, and they could pay me what they wanted to pay me, which was good because I got a little more. But more importantly, it meant that I could organize things. I said, "Okay, we have a compliance problem? No problem. We don't dispense prescriptions, we dispense medications," so 100 percent filled prescriptions. So now compliance is not an issue.

We knew everyone's relatives. Thank goodness they were all related. If someone had an abnormal test result, we didn't send a letter. We called the police. And the police would go out to their house, knock on their door and say, "Go to the clinic; the doctor needs to see you; I'll give you a ride."

So we had 100 percent compliance insofar as compliance could be an issue. *Yet nobody got better!* Nobody responded to the medications! *These patients had their medications, we dispensed the medications, we made sure they took the medication, and people were not getting better!* Now I was really, really bent. I was a little panicky. I had confirmed again that what the medical world told me simply wasn't the truth. It wasn't because they were poor or non-compliant. It's because this "medicine" stuff simply doesn't work.

So, I was assigned the goal of achieving 100 percent immunization on the Indian reservation. We documented every last little kid in the tribe. We talked to all the mothers, and the mothers acted how you'd expect. Some said, "I don't know if I want my kid to be immunized. It looks pretty painful and gruesome to me, and I don't think I want his spirit disturbed like that." The Chippewa Indians are very peaceful and calm people, and of course I was very convincing—I sold books door to door to get through Harvard, after all. So I talked to these women and explained things to them, encouraged them. We gave them free rides and all kinds of stuff, and our clinic received the highest immunization rate; <u>98 percent immunization rate!</u>

The Lethal Dose

I was patting myself on the back when I received another cassette in the mail. I popped the cassette in, and I listened to it. This was 1985, and the cassette said, *"The only cases of polio in North America, Central America and South America, the only cases of polio are exclusively from the vaccine. <u>The only way to get polio if you live in the United States, Central America, or South America, is to get vaccinated with the polio vaccine</u>."*

You can imagine my reaction. I wasn't there to give kids polio and lie to their mother's faces. That was not my intention at all. Something was (and is) wrong with all of this! And of course you can't get further information from anybody. I wanted to say, "Excuse me? We're giving kids polio? You know, I don't think that's right!" There was nobody to call. After all, it was the government that set the immunization goals, and the police were giving rides to the clinic. We even had a list of kids who needed shots. Some were tribal members that did not live on the reservation. Whenever they appeared on the reservation, we were alerted, and the police appeared at the mother's door to provide transportation. The police and government were all in on it. There was nobody to call.

Then there was the other problem. I returned to work, and the executive director of the clinic said, "Dr. Daniels, you've done a great job. You are so effective; you have turned things around. Do you realize this reservation was going to erupt in riots over dissatisfaction over health care? And now we have Indians coming back to the reservation to *get* health care."

Dr. Jennifer Daniels

We even had white men who wanted to come to the clinic to receive health care *because they heard about people getting better*. Of course we couldn't take care of them because administratively we were set up to just give free care. We couldn't issue bills, and we weren't allowed to do this, we weren't allowed to do that. So the whites were angry because, "Hey, this is from my federal dollars too. It's my tax dollars paying for this clinic, so what do you mean I can't come here for care?"

So when people showed up in my office and were having side effects from their drugs, I had no problem stopping the drugs. I said, "Man, I don't think it's working for you. We need to change. We need to switch." So if nothing else, at least I had that flexibility where other doctors did not. Now the doctors in town weren't saying that; they were just continuing these drugs and killing the people. Patients and doctors do not see side effects as a warning. If they did, a lot of deaths could be avoided.

People were even leaving the Marshville Clinic to come to the clinic I managed on the reservation. Marshfield Clinic is a very prestigious, very large clinic, with hundreds of doctors hyper-specialized, and big, big bucks rolling in.

So from my perspective, it wasn't like I cured anyone. I saw several patients a day, and I could see for myself that no one was getting better from their medications. Consider their medications and side effects though, and what a patient is likely to see is that with the other doctor they felt like crap and worse crap because of the medications.

The Lethal Dose

With, me they felt a lot better because I helped them avoid side effects rather than pushing the drug further. So relatively speaking, if a patient came to see me, they were going to feel better than before and be a little more able to get on with their lives instead of feeling totally debilitated.

Through cutting them back or taking them off certain medications, patients were able to go to work, to still play baseball on the baseball team because they had energy, or whatever it may be that they consider "better." On the other hand, a doctor in town would leave them on horrible medicines, high dosages, etc. So the patients couldn't do much. As such, I didn't have much competition.

With this lack of flexibility seen in many doctors, a doctor who's sticking to the Standard of Care without deviation, patients are predictably going to die. The death rate I calculated, or observed in my medical practice, was about 4 deaths per year for a one-doctor practice. That's 4 deaths per year per family practice doctor, if you stick to the Standard of Care.

In my practice while sticking to the Standard of Care, I observed that people weren't getting better. In fact, they were getting worse. I'd send patients to a specialist thinking that the specialist would take a look at my therapy and say, "You know, Dr. Daniels, let's change this, change that..." I assumed that the specialist would recommend something that would make the patient better. They came back, and the specialist had made recommendations, *and invariably the patients got worse*!

Obviously this is an issue. I could see my patient getting worse, so I tell them, as any caring person would, "Excuse me, Mr. Jones, I see that you're getting worse. Maybe we can send you back to the specialist, or maybe we can change something here." And I was absolutely floored when patients would say, "Oh, no, I've seen the specialist. This is what he wants, and I'm going to continue with it." Sometimes I would send them back to the specialist and he would give them another change. Guess what happened? It made them *even worse off*!

The last straw for me was one particular patient. She was an extremely nice nurse in her mid-30s. She was married, and she had a little kid around 18 months old. This would be a happy family except that she had lupus. So she came to see me, and I said, "Well you have lupus. Let me send you to the specialist and see what he recommends."

So I sent her to a specialist, who recommended high doses of steroids with a taper, which is standard lupus care. So I followed exactly what he said, and then she had a flare. I sent her back to the specialist and three months later, she was dead.

This really was a breaking point. How does this happen? A 36-year-old lady walks into my office alive, and she's dead three months later? Something I did must have led

The Lethal Dose

to that death. I called up the specialist and told him she was dead. The conversation went like this.

I said, "You know that nice lady that I sent to you?"

"Oh, yeah, yeah, yeah."

I said, "Well, she's dead."

"Oh, really?"

I said, "Yes."

"Well, did you do everything I told you?"

I said, "Yes, I did. I did exactly what you told me."

He said, "Oh, well, then don't worry, *no problem. No problem.*"

Me: "No problem? The patient is dead. Can we get together a different game plan for the next patient?"

He says, "Oh, no, no, no, not necessary. As long as we're *doing everything according to the Standard of Care*, if the patients die it's not anything to worry about. Patients will die."

For me, that was simply not acceptable. That just kind of broke everything loose. I then had to confront the very real fact in my mind that what I was doing was contributing to peoples' death. Honestly I could not sleep for months.

So nobody investigated. Fine. Nobody sued. Fine.

Even if they had sued, *they would not have gotten a single penny!* Not a penny, because *malpractice is defined as "deviation from the Standard of Care."* If you <u>do not deviate from the Standard of Care</u>, you are *totally immune, there is no malpractice*! Even if the care provided caused the death!!

This type of thought process, the health care system in general, and my role in particular, had me worried.

The Lethal Dose

PAYING THE PRICE FOR HELPING THE COMMUNITY

Let's move ahead in time. At some point along the way, I became extremely open-minded. I told myself, "Okay, health is not just a drug thing, not just a food thing; *it's a community thing*." So I started looking around and decided, "Let's get rid of this drug violence." My mother had to walk by the drug dealers on her way to the office and they were not being very nice to her. I reasoned that drug dealers, like any other species, needed a habitat. Destroy their habitat and they would leave. I started by getting drug dens demolished and streets paved and sidewalks repaired. It worked. Later, I got affordable family homes built, and the neighborhood was on a roll.. Really it was like a movement. It was just incredible how this little block of the ghetto in Syracuse, New York, started looking pretty suburban.

A bond issue came along where it was proposed to borrow $30 million in the name of school renovations to finance the renovation of six buildings, three of which were private and the kids would never be allowed access to. The bond required that the city repay $45 million! I said, "That makes no sense. Why are we going to spend money from the educational budget to renovate private citizens' businesses and repay $45 million? That's nonsense!"

I lobbied, and the government said, "Oh, go practice medicine." Afterward, I crunched the numbers, and this and that, and I lobbied some more, and it didn't do any good.

So I said to myself, "Come on, I know how to do this. I have an MBA! A bank has got to make this loan, right? We can't pay back a loan the bank won't make, now can we?"

A guy on the inside managed to give me a copy of the bank letter of credit. A letter of credit is basically a note from the bank that lists reasons they won't keep a promise to lend you money. This letter was 21 pages long! So I had plenty of reasons to pick from. I read it and picked out all the things that were true in terms of why the bank should *not* lend the money. I got about 300 people to write letters and say, "We are not in favor of the project, and if our government borrows the money we don't want them to pay it back!"

So I packaged these 300 letters plus a cover letter. This cover letter basically said, "You will never see your money, and if you try and collect you will have to use draconian tactics that will make your Third World activities look genteel." When I sent this off to the bankers, they made modifications to the project that killed it.

Yet, the governor had already been bribed. I didn't know that. So, the governor dropped the dime and called the licensing board and said, "This doctor does not need a license."

The Lethal Dose

They took away my license. I'm also on two "Do Not Employ" lists, and I'm also on the Terrorist Watch List which is why I'm currently in Panama.

There were points where it got pretty terrifying. You're in your home, the government has done this to you, and you don't know when the government is going to come next. Then, there is the occasional knock on the door with yet another letter of summons or telling you what additional privilege of citizenship you no longer have. I had no idea what they might do next. I didn't know if they were going to abduct me, if they're going to torture me, lock me up, etc. In my case, the charges kept changing.

They don't even have to charge you with anything. If there are no charges, you don't even know what the *penalty* is. You don't even know where all this ends. You ask yourself, "Can they *take everything I own?* Can they dismember me one fingernail at a time? *Is there a death penalty* here? Is it 20 years, is it 5 years?" I couldn't even make plans because I did know if I would make it across town without government intervention.

I just needed a little peace of mind. I just needed to relax. *I needed another country.* I tell you this, not for your sympathy. I just want you to realize what your doctor would be facing if he took a holistic view toward your health or deviated from the Standard of Care.

So I went shopping for countries, and I picked Panama. It turned out to be an extremely enchanting place to live.

Dr. Jennifer Daniels

The whole thing has been a wonderful experience, even outside of having a bit less to worry about. When I arrived, I couldn't speak the language at all, and I would highly recommend it to people travelling to stay someplace where you don't speak the language. You are *totally immune to the propaganda being blared all over the place.* All the negative news, you don't see. All you *see and experience is the actual people* and how nice and how kind they are. So for me, until I mastered a fair amount of Spanish, I was really in a state of euphoria.

Now that I have a little bit of Spanish, I can see a negative headline, but now I realize that is just conditioning propaganda. The people here are absolutely fabulous. They are wonderful. I live in a Panamanian neighborhood, and my neighbors take it as a badge of pride that a gringo lives in their neighborhood. At the time of writing, I've been here for four years.

Still, the well-deserved retaliation from my own government during my attempts to help patients surprised me. I realize now that the worse offense is to interfere with the activities of government. A patient that heals or a governor that cannot deliver on a bribe cannot be tolerated.

If I had *just* lost my license, it would be no big deal. I could go sell insurance or something to continue surviving. Yet when you are put on the Do Not Employ list and then you are put on the Terrorist Watch? Well that's another story.

The Lethal Dose

As per the Do Not Employ list, I cannot be employed by anyone who receives government grants of any kind, and I cannot be employed by anyone who has a contract with anyone who has a government grant of any kind. As you might imagine, that means I can barely work anywhere in the United States.

If I had been a high school dropout, I would have more job opportunities than if I was a doctor who lost their license. Of course, other doctors know this also, and this is what they are up against. This is what your doctor is facing should he or she refuse to murder or try to heal you.

The only way to get off the Do Not Employ list is to get my license back in New York state, but New York state has a license repatriation rate of less than 10 percent. Even if it were possible, it would take several years.

As per the Do Not Fly list, I get the four SSSSs on my ticket, when I buy a ticket. I don't fly anymore because it's too much stress, but I would go up to the counter and I hand the ticket agent my passport. The worker scans the passport—I was in the United States and I forget what airport—and she looks at the passport and then calls the supervisor. I could hear her whisper, "What do I do, what do I do?" And the supervisor looks at me, looks at the computer screen, and I guess they assess the level of threat. They say, "Don't worry, issue the ticket. They'll take care of it at the other end."

So she issues the ticket. I look at it, and sure enough, the four SSSSs. I go the place where you check in before you do the weapons check and the electronic stuff. They say, "Excuse me, step over here." Then you hear on the loudspeaker: "Female Security, Emergency! Female Security Emergency!" I know it's about to be a heap of trouble for me, even if everything does work out.

Then you get this committee that assembles, and it just becomes an ordeal. It's very traumatic because you don't know if you're going to be abducted, turned away, or anything else. This happens every time I want to fly. This is what your doctor is facing if he steps out of line.

The Lethal Dose

MAKING MONEY IN THE HOSPITAL, DEAD OR ALIVE

The media are the ones who are spreading the flu virus. Not in the sense that they literally go out and spread the virus, but they are giving people the flu because people buy into the idea that *they already have it, so any symptom they have they attribute to the flu.*

It's the *attribution* that's important. For example, if a person's immune system heals them, they attribute that healing to the doctor. If they get worse, they attribute that to their immune system. *It's all about attribution.* So if you have someone attributing any little symptom—a sneeze, a sniffle, a headache—to the flu, then what would have been just a normal 5-minute headache or a one-day tummy virus six months ago, now it's the flu!

Here's an example. Two other couples, nice people, gringos, were in a restaurant with us, and we'd just ordered. And the guy at the end of the table, a really nice guy, whips out his hand sanitizer and wipes it on his hands and generously offers a hand sanitizer to everyone around the table. Now my husband of course, he lives with me so he knows the drill, and he's heard all the stuff. Still, he's not as discreet as I might be. I would have taken the hand sanitizer and passed it on. My husband says,

Dr. Jennifer Daniels

"That hand sanitizer isn't helping you! Ask my wife! Jennifer, tell him!"

So the hand sanitizer is an attribution. Because what we're really trying to get rid of is *some deadly germ* that's going to kill us. But *what deadly germ is killing everybody?*

Answer: there are <u>*two deadly germs*</u> that account for 63,000 deaths a year, every year, in the United States. That's MRSA (methicillin resistant staph) and C.difficile.

Now here's what you need to know about these two deadly germs: the *only way* to get them is to be *exposed to antibiotics. You must take an antibiotic, and when you take the antibiotic those germs actually evolve and are created on your body.* So I can't get MRSA. I can get MRSA by kissing my husband just because he has it. MRSA is going to dissipate, and that would be the end of it.

So this guy, by using a hand sanitizer, is actually ignoring the true hazard–antibiotics. The hand sanitizers mostly contain alcohol which, for many reasons, is ineffective.

You can't really get these or die from them unless you take an antibiotic. It's that complicated. You're a human being, and you have skin. On the skin is an organism called staph. (The full name is Staphlycoccus Aureus, a common bacterium.) Staph germs are sensitive to just about any and every antibiotic. If you put an antibiotic on your skin or in your body, that staph germ then takes on a plasmid, which you could compare to antivirus soft-

The Lethal Dose

ware, and that plasmid keeps the staph germ from dying when exposed to antibiotics. The more antibiotics you expose the staph germs to, the more protective software, so to speak, they pick up. Then the staph germ becomes really strong, really robust.

Then you go to the hospital, and what happens at the hospital? They stick you with a needle, an IV, and then this bacteria gets in through the skin through the very hole they stuck you with. *That's* when it becomes deadly.

So you can have these deadly flesh-eating bacteria, but as long as it's sitting on top of your skin, it is harmless. It becomes deadly when the hospital puts a hole in your skin, either with an IV a urinary catheter or any of the many other tubes that are inserted at hospitals.

That is all easy enough to understand, but let's keep on this linear path. What happens if you *stop* taking antibiotics of all kinds? The staph germ apparently is spending a lot of energy maintaining this protective software, and it jettisons it, and it goes back to becoming an everyday, harmless staph germ.

When you take antibiotics, the staph germs *supercharge themselves* by *taking on plasmids* that protect them from being killed by the antibiotic, but the plasmids also make *this mild-mannered staph into a huge, ferocious, flesh-eating bacteria.*

If you stop the antibiotics, then the staph germs jettison these plasmids, and at the rate of about 30 percent per month. People who are positive for this deadly bacteria will actually revert to being negative.

This is why we see all the dangers of staph infections in hospitals, nursing homes, and other medical settings. It's the puncture wound from the needles or surgeries after the prescribing of antibiotics that actually cause the problems. Interestingly, 37 percent of all the meat sold in the United States is *laced* with this particular resistant staph. This isn't the harmless staph on our skin, it's the *deadly* staph, *the flesh-eating staph that kills everybody*. So if you go to a store and you buy a hot dog, there's a 47 percent chance you're also *eating* this deadly bacteria with your hot dog. Guess how it got there? T*he farmer fed antibiotics to the hog. Hand sanitizers offer absolutely no protection in this regard.*

As the antibiotics fed to the cow, pig, chicken, etc., and then it is ingested by you. These antibiotics are actually *causing this plasmid to develop.* Not only are we confronted with issues from the medical field, but our own food industry is just as likely to cause our health problems. It's apparent that there's something extremely wrong going on.

You can also eat meat that doesn't have the MRSA deadly bacteria on it, and it just has the antibiotic. The antibiotic gets into your system, and *your body goes on to develop its own deadly bacteria as a result of exposure to antibiotics.* So we

The Lethal Dose

have people who are wearing gloves in the hospitals, wearing masks, wearing gowns, and they are bringing into the person's room *a meal the doctor ordered that is laced with the deadly bacteria that will ultimately kill them.* There are certainly not natural organic or grass-fed meats in hospitals.

It's a "cooperative effort." The hospital *knows* that if they keep feeding you the hospital food, you're going to be sick. They know you're going to stay sicker and sicker, *and they make more money*! The average person probably doesn't realize that if you go to the hospital and get discharged alive, the hospital will collect $10,000 on average. That's *IF* you get discharged alive. Whether you pay for it, insurance pays for it, or the government pays for it, they'll get this money somewhere.

More surprisingly, if you go to the hospital and you're discharged to the morgue, the hospital collects an average amount of $45,000. Doesn't matter who pays it: government, insurance, family, your estate. Either way, they'll get this money. What does this tell you? *Going into the hospital is really treacherous for you. Once they murder you, and collect the $45,000, there is no investigation, no criminal charges, not even malpractice because it was done using the Standard of Care.*

As I mentioned earlier, when your doctor follows the *Standard of Care,* as he is taught to do all throughout medical school, then he is covered and protected from possible lawsuits. Your doctor has full <u>immunity</u>. He has a shield of almost Biblical proportions. It's insane how impermeable this armor really is. If you recommend a vegetable, you step outside of that shield. If you recommend, "Excuse me, maybe we could stop the antibiotics," then that's it. You're a goner; you lose everything. You lose your license, the insurance companies won't pay, and the patients call you a quack. It's simply devastating trying to actually help people.

PRESCRIPTION DRUGS

Let's talk about prescription medications a bit. At some point, I started to figure out that *the less prescription medications I gave patients, lower doses spaced out longer, the better they actually recovered.* Then I realized that taking them off prescriptions completely helps patients get better even quicker.

People would come in. I would size them up. People actually started flying in from California, New York, even Europe and Canada to come see me because they couldn't find a doctor in between who would explain this to them in English. A new patient would show up from wherever, and I'd say, "Look here, you're on 10 drugs. Right now, I can tell you that if you stop these five, you won't even notice. If anything, you'll feel better. We've got five more left after that. Now with these five, you can only stop them if you're really going to do what I'm telling you to do. Here's what I want you to do…"

Then I'd tell them how much I want them to drink, what I want them to drink, what they're supposed to eat, how many times you're supposed to poop. I'd say, "Can you do that?" If they agreed to follow my directions, I'd tell them that it's time to get off all their medications.

Some would say, "Oh, doctor, that's a whole lot you're asking me. You know, I can only do two of those five things."

I'd say, "Okay, fine, you do two of them, and we'll stop two or three of these drugs here. We'll just kind of ease you off." So that's what I did.

The drugs aren't keeping anyone alive. If those five drugs were stopped all at once, then the person will suddenly go back to feeling the way they felt before the drugs were started. Maybe they were having a headache or they had pain or something, and there's a reason the person was uncomfortable or started taking the drugs. So if they just stop the drugs and do nothing, then the symptoms that were there that caused them to go on the drugs in the first place will recur.

I'm not advocating anything, but I've had more than one person tell me, "Dr. Daniels, I felt so bad I just wanted to die. So I stopped all of my drugs, and I got better." So I cannot sit here and honestly tell you that it's dangerous to stop all your drugs. At the same time, I can't practice medicine and tell anyone, "Oh, stop your drugs." *We have laws in place that favor speaking out in favor of drugs.*

If a doctor says to someone, "You know what? Your drug benefit is all in your brain. Why don't you just toss them out the window and be happy?" Well… that kind of discussion is not allowed. That doesn't mean there aren't alternatives, though. Prescription drugs are a money

The Lethal Dose

making venture, and there's a lot of misinformation on all sides.

Let's discuss package inserts, which are packets of information on medications. A package insert is written in 7 point type. Often it is even smaller than this. There's a reason for this mode of publication: *the average doctor or patient that takes medicines can't read that small of type.*

Within that tiny text, the package insert lists all the dangers and hazards of the medicine. This is information that isn't even mentioned when pharmaceutical companies go to doctors and market their product. Even if your doctor did know about this information, this isn't the type of information the drug companies would tell a patient in the patient information handouts.

This package insert explains the *true death rate from the medication*. For example, there's this new drug out called Brillianta*, which thins your blood and help protects you against heart attacks. Well, there's a four percent death rate from that drug! It's only a 3.6 percent death rate from heart attack. If everyone who did not take the drug had a heart attack instead, the death rate at the end of the year would only be 3.6 percent. Less than if one took the drug. So, taking the drug that prevents heart attack is more deadly than *having* the heart attack. Of course, if you don't read it or never even receive the package insert, then you don't get that information. You do not know that you have to have a 103% chance of a heart attack in order to benefit from the drug.

It remains a mystery. So, you rely on your doctor and the Standard of Care. Most of patients never know that they're taking a gamble by taking prescriptions given by their doctors.

One of the scariest parts of this whole package insert deal is that *there are doctors who are prescribing drugs who have never read the package insert themselves.* Why? The drug is detailed to them *without* a package insert, and they don't often demand that they get it before prescribing a new drug. Another reason is that most package inserts are written in 7-point type, which is illegible to most Doctors and patients.

A third reason is that doctors attend these continuing medical education (CME) courses that tell them how to use the drugs. Many doctors are relying on the information taught at these conferences when they prescribe medicine. Normally it sounds like more education is a good idea, but everything they hear at those CME courses is paid for by the drug companies themselves. Drug companies, hospitals or insurance companies literally pay each speaker at these symposiums. So, if you have a doctor education conference, this is how you make money on it. Every speaker is free because the drug company compensates them and pays their travel and hotel. The drug companies pay to rent booths. Doctors pay them to attend because it is a mandatory condition of keeping their license. You, the conference organizer, only have to pay for the venue and marketing costs. If you work out a deal with the hotel, they may give you the conference space

The Lethal Dose

free if a certain number of attendees rend rooms there. Setting up these conferences is very profitable. That's what we call "continuing your medical education."

All of this is important because as many as 107,000 patients die from properly prescribed drugs each year in the United States. This *is* murder. Every doctor has seen a drug kill patients. The doctor knows if he or she keeps following the same protocols, patients will die. Yet doctors do not dare stop it, because it's the Standard of Care. <u>So, if the person is doing something and they know that death is going to result when they do it, then "murder" might be a reasonable term.</u> We're effectively having people take pills voluntarily that can kill them. Let's return to the topic of package inserts in a moment.

Obviously, you can understand why you need to read the package insert if at all possible. The thing about this is that your doctor doesn't even have the package insert for themselves. You'd think it would come along with the medications samples and information on the medication, but it's really not that common for doctors to be able to give you this information. As a doctor, I had to tell the drug companies that they couldn't leave me a medication sample without the darn package insert!

So if you needed or wanted to see the package inserts, you would have to do one of two things. One, go to the pharmacist that dispensed the drugs and demand the package inserts. A lot of times, you'll have to be really stern and aggressive about this. You literally have to demand this from most pharmacies. They have no real incentive to dig this out for you, especially once you've already paid them. Just refuse to leave until you get the package insert.

The other method of getting package inserts is good ol' Google. This will take a little effort on your part but if you have home internet, it is quicker than going to the pharmacist. Go to Google and search for the name of the drug, followed by "package insert." At least two of the choices on the first page search results will actually have the package insert. If you are going to take prescription medication, be sure to read these package inserts even if you have to use a magnifying glass just to see the text.

The Lethal Dose

DRUG TOXICITY AND THE TRUTH ABOUT THE PHARMCUTICAL DRUG MODEL

So we know that prescription drugs are full of toxicity and other issues, yet why is it that doctors don't acknowledge this regularly? Pretty simple. If they did, they'd be where I am today: sitting in Panama on the Terrorist Watch List. When I was being persecuted, harassed by the state, I thought, "What did I do wrong? I treated this patient and he got better, and now they are taking my license away because he got better without drugs." I didn't quite understand it yet.

And so one doctor said, "You did *what*!? You gave a patient a *choice*?!" As if this were some outlandish thing to do. As if their life and the way they live it shouldn't have been discussed and decided by them! So that's one thing. Doctors are never to give the patient a choice.

Here's a true example of something else that I experienced directly when I was a resident at a hospital where a patient had been overdosed on heparin. Heparin thins your blood, and if you take too much, you'll bleed to death. That's all you need to know really. And so I had prescribed heparin. The nurse erroneously gave eight

Dr. Jennifer Daniels

times the drug at four times the rate. She had overdosed him. She realized her error after four hours, in which of course she gave closer to 30-hours worth of medicine. So she comes to me just trembling, "Oh, my God, how can we save this patient's life?" She tells me the situation!

I'm sitting next to the attending physician in charge of the patient, and I'm just the grunt, right? I said, "Okay, look, do this, stop it immediately. Immediately stop the drug. We've got to check his urine for blood, check this, check him to see if he's bleeding anywhere." I had the whole thing ready to go in place.

The senior doctor—I'm in training, a resident, and this is a doctor who's earning big bucks, a cardiologist—he yells, "Don't you *ever*, don't you *ever* stop a drug! *Never* stop a drug, *especially* on my patient!" He went into a tirade.

Now, I was trembling. So I said, "Well, okay, Dr. So and So, what do you want him to have?" And I took out that order sheet, and I wrote down the order of exactly what he wanted the patient to have, exactly how much. I put a little X there, handed the sheet of instructions to him. He signed it. I couldn't believe he signed it.

I then handed the signed order to the nurse, and she was white as a sheet, because she knew as I knew the patient was getting a lethal dose.

53

The Lethal Dose

So, she went to her supervisor and explained the whole thing to the supervisor. The supervisor said—this really happened—"Is that Dr. So and So's valid signature?"

And she said, "Yes."

"Then it's your duty to follow orders."

I mean, if her job description was giving lethal injections on death row, it would look about the same. The nurse, afraid for her job went in and *continued that drug, exactly the concentration, just as the doctor ordered*! As shocked as I was that the doctor signed the orders, I was more disturbed that the nurse did not resign on the spot. Murder is a high price to pay to keep a job. Many health care workers knowingly pay this price every day.

Predictably, five hours later, the patient started bleeding from every hole he owned. And they had to transfuse 26 units of blood and call in the blood from all around Philadelphia to keep him from dying. This guy was a dentist, in the peak of his work career. Ultimately he lost his eyesight, was permanently blind, because he bled into his eyeballs.

Needless to say, the hospital settled out of court. But, I am sure that victim would have preferred to have his eyesight and his career. So you ask, "Why don't doctors *acknowledge* it!?"

There I was. I *was* acknowledging it. What happened? There were so many mechanisms in place to over – ride any attempt to interfere with the lethal dose. I ordered the lethal dose stopped; I was ordered not to. I refused to sign the lethal orders; the senior doctor signed it. The nurse didn't want to give it; she was intimidated by her supervisor. The system as well as the individuals surrounding me, conspired to be sure the patient got the lethal dose. The only power I had was to refuse to be a part of it.

Just for the record, I did hand in my resignation first thing the next business day. It was declined and I was given special permission to speak up or refuse to give lethal doses of drugs.

So doctors are conditioned *not to acknowledge*. Whatever the problem, whatever the issue, the drug is *not* the problem. If a doctor discontinues drugs because he believes the drugs are harming someone, that's an express train to losing his license, as you can see in my example.

It's bad enough that doctors are too scared for their licenses and willing to basically commit murder, but this is all aided by the drug companies as well as hospital policies. There's a very obvious and specific model that goes into pharmaceutical

The Lethal Dose

The big picture can be simplified into the easy to understand steps below:

1) The drug company patents a drug
2) The drug company determines the minimum lethal dose
3) The drug company sets the recommended dose at a level that is HIGHER than the lethal dose
4) The doctors are expected to (and do) prescribe the lethal dose so they (the hospital and the drug companies) can sell the maximum amount of the drug possible, and therefore earn the most profits possible.
5) Hospitals agree to be a place where dangerous drugs can be administered and monitored
6) The hospital makes certain that insurance is in place.
7) Everyone gets paid when the patient finally dies.

That is the medical model we live with today. The Doctor gives a drug at lethal doses until the patient dies. Ideally, the patient's driver's license has the donor box checked. The medical industry then harvests the organs for additional profits. *That is the strategy*. The strategy is not "heal and bill." It's "kill to bill."

So with that model in place, you can literally make garlic deadly. The drug industry has determined a lethal dose for Turmeric. Look for a turmeric analog soon. So the drugs are designed to be lethal, and that's why 107,000 people die every year from *properly prescribed drugs*. It is actually designed that way.

You can go to my website and watch that video, "Murder by Medicine is No Accident." It explains how the drugs are *actually designed to kill*. I actually analyze a drug, explain to you how the drug is being marketed, what the package insert says. The package insert just tells the doctors to *prescribe this drug until the undertaker arrives*.

I'm putting it in plain English so you can understand it, but it says that basically, *"This drug causes liver damage, prescribe it until the patient is urinating black and defecating gray."* At that point, you have irreversible liver damage, and the person is basically dead. So *this is the point* at which the package insert instructs the doctor to stop the drugs.

This is our medical system.

Now when we step out and make the decision to remove these drugs from our personal healing strategy and daily lives, we're left with plenty of questions. One question is, "How do I detox?" Well, the only way to reverse drug toxicity is to not take drugs. That's number one. So if you're trying to reverse drug toxicity by taking drugs, the drugs you take to reverse it are going to cause their own toxicity. So number one, stop the drugs. Number two: increase your water.

The Lethal Dose

Number three, increase your intake of organic, but, honestly, foraged wild vegetation that grows around your house. If they'll let you put a chicken in the back yard, eat the chicken, but revert to natural food.

Then you have to clean out your bowels. If you're into colonics, do colonics. Do enemas. Have more bowel movements. Vitality Capsules will help with this product (find it online at http://vitalitycapsules.com/vitality-capsules-are-made-of-whole-herbs-packed-in-veggie-caps). We'll talk more about detoxing, how to poop more, and Vitality Capsules later on.

Even before my license was taken away, I was substituting natural remedies for prescription drugs. I was using my prescription pad to write down recipes. I'd say, "Okay, you can't give up your cheese, huh? Hmm. Here, put these in your blender and blend it up. It tastes just like cheese. And this way you can heal, get your cheese flavor, and you'll do fine."

I had to teach myself a lot of the natural remedies I use. I had become extremely ill at one point. While pregnant with my first child. I became vegetarian. When you look in the back of most vegetarian magazines, you see a bunch of natural healing books they advertise, and I would buy these quite often. As this continued, one thing led to another, and I would try things out.

It's probably no surprise, but 90 percent of the stuff does not work. Anyway, I would try it out on myself and try it on some family members, and whatever worked, I would stick with. If it didn't work? Forget it! No sense spending time on methods that don't give any real results.

Through testing and developing, I managed to gain a pretty reliable repertoire of recipes and natural remedies that worked better than the prescription drugs I had been trained to use. I honestly didn't need to use antibiotics anymore. There was no point in prescribing narcotics, not even the non-steroidal arthritis pills. After learning about natural remedies the smart way, there are just so many drugs you don't *need* anymore. It was just so exhilarating to be able to just *write on a prescription pad*, "Go to the grocery store, get this, use it this way. Drink this much. You'll be better in 24 hours." Not only was this way more effective than those annoying Standard of Care guidelines, but I didn't even have to deal with any after-hour calls because the person was having NO side effects. *This meant I could be a solo practice doctor, provide 24 hour call and still get sleep.*

DOCTORS ARE HOLOGRAMS

There's a point that people need to understand. You take the pills. You can decide not to take the pills. The point is this:

People need to stop asking permission for things they already have the right to do.

That is the crux of the matter. You have the right to stop your medications. *Your doctor cannot murder you without your total permission and cooperation.* Your doctor is nothing more than a *hologram*. That's all he is. Let me repeat: your doctor is a hologram. *You* need to pay your health insurance premium each month. You need to get the prescription from the doctor. *You* need to go fill it. *You* need to get the pill, and *you* need to put it in your mouth. *The doctor cannot kill you without your total and complete cooperation.* In fact, you do almost all of the work for them.

So if you understand that your doctor is a hologram, like your TV set, you just turn off the button. You're in control here. But you need to understand that he is just a hologram. You are the one allowing this hologram to influence you in ways that harm you. *You* are perceiving this hologram as real. But it's not.

Dr. Jennifer Daniels

Likewise, your hands are kind-of tied with your relatives and loved ones. If they are trusting of the hologram, it is not really in your power to turn off the switch. You can get the package inserts and try to explain to them what it says, but in the end, it's their decision. So what I do with my mother, and my mother is 81, I say, "Ma, you got that drug from the doctor, and I don't think it's a good idea to take it."

She says, "Well, I'm your mother, and I'm going to take this drug!!"

I say, "Okay, Mom. I'll tell you what, Mom–if you have a problem, let me know, and if you don't want to let me know, then here are some things you might want to try just in case."

And so, invariably, Mom ends up stopping the drug within two weeks because she can't take the side effects.

I'll tell you one really pitiful thing that happened. My mom broke her hip, ended up in the rehab, and they put her on a painkiller after surgery. That all sounds very reasonable, doesn't it?

They said, "Now, Ms. Daniels, you take this pain pill every single day before physical therapy, and don't wait to get pain because your physical therapy is important."

As most people would, she says, "Okay, okay."

The Lethal Dose

So I call her every day, because I'm here in Panama, and I am on the terrorist watch list. I can't exactly go there and help her out at a moment's notice.

One day, I call and she says, "You know, I am wetting my pants. I had an accident. I didn't get to the bathroom in time, and I peed all over myself. But the orderly was really nice, and he gave me diapers."

I said, "Oh god, Mom."

So then Mom says, "But you know, I'm getting a little forgetful, a little forgetful here, and I guess I'm getting... I'm 80 years old." This was last year.

I said, "All right, Mom, what drug are you taking?"

She says, "Well, I'm taking this pain pill."

So I look up the very common pain pill, and wouldn't you know what I found out? Doesn't that drug *cause you to piss your pants and forget everything*! It's right there in the package insert.

So I call Mom back and I say, "Mom, that drug is making you piss your pants and forget everything!"

Mom was shocked. "No! What am I going to do?"

I said, "Mom, I think you need to refuse the drug!"

Dr. Jennifer Daniels

She said the same thing many people say: "Well, can I ask my doctor to not prescribe that?"

I said, "Mom. Get a grip. Refuse the drug, Mom. Spit it out. Toss it on the ground. Flush it. Whatever. Just don't take it!"

So Mom felt it necessary to engage the nurse in a conversation. I'm famous back in Syracuse, which makes her the doctor's mother. So she mentioned that she didn't think that she should take a pain pill and she wanted the doctor to stop the pain pill. It worked, and it immediately was done, done, done. She no longer took the drug. If you are not the parent of a doctor, it may not go as well for you.

Mom became the celebrity of the rehab ward. She's sitting at the table with these two old ladies, and everyone's 80 years old, and this one lady says, "You know, I'm wearing diapers, and it's so embarrassing. I can't remember things either and I don't really know what to do." My mother piped up, "Well, I don't take that pain pill anymore, and it was making me wet my pants and I stopped it. I just couldn't be *bothered* wearing diapers and having my children run my life!"

The next day Mom overheard the nurse offering this patient a pain pill, and the patient said, "Oh, no, thank you. I'm cutting back."

The Lethal Dose

So many people are wearing diapers because of the medication their doctors are giving them according to the Standard of Care!

You may assume that there are millions of people in nursing homes and hospitals that are literally being kept alive by prescription drugs because their bodies become dependent on them, but this isn't true. What's happening is that they're kept in a drugged state so they can be farmed and exploited at a rate of $10,000 to $30,000 a month. Those people—without their drugs and with real food, if you want to call it that—would be at home managing their own homes, managing their own affairs, meddling in the lives of their children and grandchildren and great-grandchildren. They would literally be living a full life!

If my mother had not stopped those drugs, then she would be in bed, babbling to herself, and we would be wringing our hands about where to place her. I'm being completely literal here, too.

But *because she stopped those drugs,* Mom is at home. She's walking. She's talking. She's cooking. She's driving her own car, and she's got an opinion about everything. And if she doesn't agree with you, she lets you know!

What I'm trying to say is that these people who are living in nursing homes are living differently. They could all be living the way my mother is living *if they were treated differently.* So the fact that they are in a nursing home is a product of toxic foods, toxic drugs and social conditioning. The holograms and the belief in these Holograms (doctors) permit this to happen.

If you are taking drugs and having side effects, you have already started on the path to becoming one of these nursing home vegetables in a drugged state. That is how it starts.

The Lethal Dose

WRITING RECIPES ON MY PRESCRIPTION PAD

As I mentioned, I've worked hard to come up with some natural remedies and cures for a number of ailments and medical issues. As my understanding evolved, I started using my prescription pad to write recipes for people. And so I was prescribing recipes for their afflictions instead of drugs. I have written a collection of healing recipes. These are now a collection of my healing recipes. You can find them as 4 eBooks on Vitalitycapsules.com. Now many people are skeptical of natural cures, and while I can understand that sentiment, I can offer you just as much experience that says the status quo just isn't working.

If you're looking for any proof that prescription drugs, vaccines, and other medical "treatments" are somehow not what they seem, then you can turn to several examples. I can tell you a few personal stories on the matter. A good one is the polio vaccine that we mentioned earlier. I recently had a woman ask me why her blood shows a very high count of polio antibodies 15 years post-vaccine and why she has mild but troubling neurological symptoms.

The thing about vaccines is that you still have antibodies and other effects 15 years later because *the vaccine gave you polio*. It may not be fatal, but *you have low-grade polio from*

Dr. Jennifer Daniels

the vaccine. All of us who received the polio vaccine, which is most of us, still have a little bit of polio. You would hope that the body would eventually flush this out, but that's not the case.

Because it was *injected into you*, it bypassed your saliva, your tonsils, the acid in your stomach, and even your liver. So your body is basically forced to play catch-up. Your whole immune system is confused about the random occurrence of something new in the system that didn't come from normal methods. It doesn't compute. Your body really is on a search and destroy mission with the polio, or other virus treated with a vaccine, and it's looking in all kinds of places it wasn't trained to look to try and find out where this virus is located. It's an overwhelming task. Your immune system can ferret out the virus, but it doesn't necessarily happen, and that's the beauty of vaccines. *One vaccine can be a lifetime of revenue to the Health Care industry.*

Now if these "vaccine preventable diseases" were actually a harmful issue, then maybe it would make sense to take the risk. Yet, the diseases the medical industry are vaccinating against are diseases that kids *are never going to get*. Unless a kid is sexually abused, there's no reason they would need to be vaccinated for hepatitis B. Even if that did happen, the chances are the rapist doesn't have hepatitis B. So why are we vaccinating our children against a whole cadre of diseases that, one, *don't exist*; and, two, the person is *not going to be exposed to*; and, three, all available

The Lethal Dose

information suggests that vaccines are just *not effective*. Even more tragic, they are *not even communicable diseases*!

Polio is spread by sewage water. Your children would have to get it by drinking sewage water. How is that a communicable disease? So we are giving vaccines for diseases that are *not even communicable*.

On the spiritual and parental aspects of this, you have a baby who's in the arms of his mother thinking, "Oh, man, I'm safe, this is my mommy, she's looking after me." Then she picks him up, takes him from her house, takes him to a place where he is tortured with needles and stabbed by strangers. You are sowing the seeds of distrust between this kid and his mother. The parents don't even realize this! You are sending this little organism the message that his mother cannot and will not protect him, and you are undermining and breaking up the family from a very young age.

I saw it in my medical practice! Kids who were not vaccinated had a different attitude towards their parents. Oh, my God, that mother-child bond was so tight it was unbelievable! None of this adolescent rebellion stuff. "This is my family, this is my mother, this is my father, I may not agree with them but by golly I love them, and I respect them, and without them I would be nothing." It's an amazing thing to behold. But vaccinate that child, and you *destroy that*. You just crush it, like throwing a wine glass on cement. At least, that's what I noticed. If I hadn't been a doctor, if I hadn't sat there and seen this... I would not have realized it.

Even more damaging than vaccines, we have antibiotics. It's easy to believe that antibiotics have been the source of cure and the saving grace needed to keep someone alive. That's just overblown optimism. Let me explain by going back to my experiences.

During my residency I was prescribing top shelf antibiotics right into peoples' veins. These patients were mainlining antibiotics. Under doctor's orders of course. I don't care what it was, whether it was cellulitis or pneumonia. It doesn't matter. With *antibiotics, the effect was not dramatic*; it was very *sluggish*. Generally the person will get better over a period of four days to a week or two or a month or never. So, I'm thinking, "Man, that was not very impressive!"

Later, I'm in family practice. So that means if the patient gets admitted to the hospital I get paid $40 bucks, and if I take care of it in the office, I get paid $90 bucks. This is not a big pay difference, but it is enough to influence my behavior. So I say to the patient, "Look, why don't we do this?" And so I used the cures in my free report, *Natural Remedies So Powerful, They Could Make Antibiotics Obsolete*. Using those remedies, people were often better in as little as *24 hours*.

Of course, I was blown away when I saw that I could use natural approaches to infection and turn the person around in 24 hours. I compared this to prescribing antibiotics for *weeks upon weeks upon weeks*, having the patients come back, and rechecking them, and changing antibiotics, and doing cultures for sensitivities—I said to myself, "I'm through; I'm not using this junk anymore!"

So did the antibiotics ever save a life? After 20 years of prescribing and witnessing the use of antibiotics, I have observed *no evidence of that*. I have to be honest, and the truth is that antibiotics account for as many as 63,000 deaths per year. The deaths from bacterial infections are almost always from the organisms created by antibiotic use. So there's no question in my mind that antibiotics are not lifesaving. A lot of those deaths are from pneumonia infections *caused by these resistant bacteria.*

If you don't employ the alternative herbal natural remedy, would the person have died if you just stopped the antibiotic and did *nothing*? I don't know. I've never done that. I stopped the antibiotic, and I've employed natural remedies, and I've seen miraculous results. These remedies are not complicated.

An example of this is an American man whose wife is from Costa Rica. He found himself in the United States when his wife fell ill. She had a respiratory problem, went to the hospital, and they gave her antibiotics. She went home, got worse, and it moved into pneumonia; she was having problems breathing. Her whole family gathered around her bed—and down here, that's bad news. So he's in the United States wringing his hands, and everyone was calling him, "Oh, help us, help us, help us."

But he says, "I'm in the United States, and I can't help you!" So he calls my husband: "Hey, I heard your wife knows something about this, and could you please help?"

So I said, "Well, what's the problem?" He said, "We think it's pneumonia, and she's fading."

I said, "Okay, here's what you do." So I told him what to do. All they needed was a common ointment you can get anywhere in the United States and overseas, any grocery store—I said, "Smear it all over her chest, every place she's got ribs just smear it. Have her drink this and move her in this position."

He listened translated the instructions into Spanish, his wife's family followed my directions, and it took two hours. Just two hours and she was breathing and feeling fine. This is even more amazing as the instructions survived translation and implementation under austere conditions.

The ointment used was made out of a lot of natural herbs. I could tell you the name, but they'd probably sue because they don't want their name being used in this context. The product is not *approved for this use*.

So that's another problem. A lot of things that could cure you and save your life are sitting in your grocery store

The Lethal Dose

disguised as something else. So in my report I tell you, "Okay, this is what it is, this is in the store, this is the name of it, go get it." These are things that cost like five bucks, or even just two bucks. So I strongly suggest that everyone go and get a copy of the report at vitalitycapsules.com while it is still free.

With antibiotics, I would say they represent one of the *biggest frauds* in the history of medicine. Out of the 808,000 annual total deaths in the hospital, 63,000 are caused by antibiotic use. That is a stunning toll for a life-saving technology.

92,000 of the 808,000 deaths by medicine happen because the doctor made a mistake. 716,000 deaths happened because the doctor accurately followed the Standard of Care. So obviously if your doctor is board-certified and following the Standard of Care, you are in *more danger* than if he's not.

Sounds a lot like medical *homicide*, doesn't it? We need to change our thinking on this topic. When you see a licensed doctor, this is really a *mass murderer* that you're looking at. When you see a patient who dies and is taking medications, that was *murder by medicine* until proven otherwise.

There needs to be an investigation! Haul out the yellow tape, man! Call CSI; get them on the case! Alert the district Attorney! This is so important if any progress is to be made. There needs to be a change in perception.

MORE ABOUT NATURAL REMEDIES

Natural remedies can replace more than just antibiotics, though. Consider menopause and hot flashes. The thing to understand about hot flashes is that they can happen at any time. If you will notice in the numerous publications and television shows on medical issues now, we have hot flashes *pre-menopause*. So if hot flashes are caused by a hormone deficiency, and a woman is still having periods, and she is getting hot flashes, the hormone imbalance theory does not work. Her hormones are balanced enough to produce periods. Her ovaries are still working, so why is she having hot flashes? The answer is: hot flashes are unrelated to hormones. Seriously, *they have nothing to do with hormones*!

What's really going on is when women stop bleeding regularly, those toxins are in your system; and you get that hot flash when your immune system is overcome and can no longer sequester the parasites and toxins. That release is perceived as a big flash. This is also why men are getting hot flashes.

If you notice, when you have that hot flash you are going sweat, and what's happening? Your body is dumping chemicals and toxins out *through your skin* that it couldn't get out through your period because you're no longer bleeding.

In other words, you're putting in so many toxins your body says, "Oh, man, if I don't get this stuff out right now, she's going to drop dead!" So then your body starts to have some hot flashes. Yet all you can think is, "Oh my, why is my body doing this to me? I'm not in menopause!" Of course, your body is trying to save your life.

So what do I do for hot flashes? I've never failed to totally eradicate the woman's hot flashes. I never, ever recommend a hormone of any kind, not even bio-identical hormones. What I recommend is that the woman start doing enemas. It's pulling more of the trash out, because if the colon is backed up into the small intestine, it's blocking the common bile duct where the liver empties its toxins into the intestine.

So if you empty your intestines out, what's going to happen is your liver is going to all of a sudden start emptying, and it's going to be able to filter blood, empty stuff, etc., and your flashes are going to go away. That's the short of how to deal with hot flashes. It doesn't take some crazy amount of hormones or other medical pills, just something you can do cheaply and easily in your own home.

Of course, to really improve the issue, obviously you have to change your diet; you have to stop eating concentrated foods that cause the flashing in the first place. You can flash by eating dried seaweed just because it's a concentrated food and it's *dry*, and your body does what? It sucks all the water from your body into your intestines to hydrate the seaweed. *Sucking water out of your blood* increases, indirectly, the level of toxins, and, boom, you have a hot flash.

So a lot of foods we think are healthy are actually contributing to our flashing. So I often help people by going over their diet, reworking that diet, go over their cleansing program, rework that, and, boom, their hot flashes are gone. Occasionally they are going to have a hot flash, but they will know, "Oh, yeah, I did that; okay, won't do that again," and no more flashes. By removing the toxins that cause the hot flashes to be necessary, you eliminate hot flashes almost entirely. While hot flashes are a form of your body detoxifying, you have enough control to give it another method of removing the toxins, which is going to be much more pleasant for you. Let the toxins leave through the colon and liver as they are supposed to rather than your skin. Otherwise, it's like you have a dinner party, and at the end of the party the guests start climbing out of the windows. Excuse me, the door is over *there*. Guide your guests to the proper exit. Next up… how to poop more!

The Lethal Dose

HOW TO POOP: VITALITY PURGING CAPSULES

I was practicing medicine, and I figured out this natural approach actually worked in some ways, right? So I was getting people healthy with diet, and things were going pretty well. But I knew people had to poop. Plenty of people would not poop; they would not have a bowel movement. And I really could not sell them on the idea of castor oil. "Oh, caster oil, quarter cup is all you need. I think it will do it for you."

Invariably, they would say, "Doc, please, no. That is why I have health insurance and come here to see you. I do not want to take castor oil. I am a grown man now."

Then I found this recipe in one of the many newsletters and books I had bought on the topic of natural cures. Then I ground it up and tried it out, and then I tried it out on my sister-in-law, and on my mother. Everyone started pooping. So they said, "Oh, this is great!"

So I ground it up at the kitchen table, and my kids packed it in capsules, and people started to buy it. So it really took off and became one of those miracle capsules. People would come by the office on Friday and say, "I need my capsules. I want to have a good weekend; I need my capsules. I don't want to be sick over the weekend."

So that's where they started. Then after I no longer practiced, I started getting them produced by a company in New Jersey. I had a quality control problem with them, so I switched to another company in the Midwest.

The capsules actually clean the gallbladder system, the liver, small intestine, and the large intestine. So it really gives a phenomenal effect besides being able to make it easy to poop. If you don't poop at all, except every two or three days, get these.

Within this product, I include ingredients such as senna, cascara sagrada, and barberry. Now there may be concerns that using capsules like this will make the body dependent on these types of ingredients to go to the bathroom, but there's a misconception here. One, the body wasn't pooping without it in the first place; that's why someone is using the capsules. Number two, the only way to train your body to poop on its own is to change the diet and change the hydration and change the activity. Yet there are two inventions that totally doomed the American culture—that's the chair and the car. Until you stop using your chair and your car, it's almost impossible to train your bowels to empty as much as they need to, to keep you disease-free. Even in other cultures though, in the 1800s when I guess we had chairs but not very many cars, *it was common to do a cleansing once a week.* Once a week the kids got castor oil to clean themselves out, or once a week people would take some kind of cathartic.

These capsules certainly fit into that program. The advantage of course is that they are convenient; you can swallow them down.

YOUR BOWELS DON'T MOVE BY THEMSELVES!

Still, I think it's a fantasy. There's no such thing as a "natural" bowel movement; your bowels *do not move by themselves*. You've got to walk, and each step you make takes the bowels and flips them over to one side, and the next step flips your bowels back. Back and forth. Your bowels are literally stimulated and moved with each step. So literally you're mechanically moving your bowels to stimulate the bowel movement. This is the major benefit of walking.

You cannot sit and hope a bowel movement will come! You've got to either move your legs there to slap those bowels around a bit, or you've got to do some belly rubbing. You've got to drink more water; you've got to stop eating stuff that's constipating.

You've got to eat more *live food*, and I'll tell you what I think live food is. Live food means you picked it out of the ground yourself; you pulled it right out of the earth. Because the problem with other so-called "live foods,"

Dr. Jennifer Daniels

they have been out of the ground so long they really can't give you that oomph, and those *enzymes that irritate* your bowels that make them move are no longer in them. So I would say that fantasy that, "Oh, don't take anything to make your bowels move because you'll train your bowels to need it," is a way to get people to *not cleanse* and to *stay sick*.

There's an old Chinese saying that after you eat you should walk 45 steps and rub your stomach in a circular direction. You can get a similar effect on the rebounder, and it's quite nice. While the actual steps aren't too important, exercise and getting your bowels moving is going to help you release your poop. And that's going to help you rid your body of toxins.

You have to have a diet that's conducive to bowel movements and activity that's conducive to it. You need to maintain them. They require your attention. As with our example on hot flashes, you can see that being able to cleanse your body is a great way to ensure there are less harmful things that can cause you to grow sick. It's really imperative that you poop!

The Lethal Dose

CONTINUING LEARNING MORE ABOUT NATURAL REMEDIES

So there quite a few indigenous people down in Panama that are open to herbs and all these things. I can't really practice as a full-time physician due to legal issues, and I don't really want to get kicked out of another country. So I obey all the laws. Still, I'm able to help many locals for free, and that's rewarding in ways money isn't.

In Panama, over the four years I've been here, I've already reversed one heart attack, kidney stones, and severe chicken pox. I live in a little casita/bungalow off the ground; it's a very steep set of steps. So if I hear the pitter patter of feet running up the steps, then I know someone needs help.

I don't charge, and I'm literally a barefoot doctor. I'm not even wearing shoes now, so I run down in my bare feet, and I help them out.

My softcover book, written with a friend of mine, is called *Do You Have the Guts to Be Beautiful?* It has a very interesting history. I wrote that book at a time of peak distress over my experience with the U.S. government. I wanted to put my knowledge in some kind of book so it would live on even if I didn't. That way, people would at least have some access to it. I didn't have the guts to name it a "healing" book, so I called it a beauty book.

People who have bought the book have lost 30 pounds; they've fixed their face so they don't need a facelift anymore; they've gotten off their medicine. Really, it's a wonderful resource that's written in a very understandable, layman, English language style. My co-author was very much into animal rights, so there's an animal rights chapter in there also. At the time I said, "Do we really need that?"

She said, "Jennifer, it's going to be a plant-based diet book!"
Nevertheless, I wrote a chapter for meat eaters on how to stay healthy while eating meat. The book is, *Do You Have the Guts to Be Beautiful?*

Past that, I offer coaching on using natural remedies to heal. I'm talking about stuff they do not teach in medical school.

If you head to my website, VitalityCapsules.com, it's called "Discovery session," and it has a program where I actually coach people individually. Click on "contact us," and we'll send you the Discovery Session link. I am really interested in passing along this type of help because I'm getting a bit older. I'm not young anymore, and this knowledge must spread.

The Lethal Dose

I'm 56, and I'm definitely on the back side of things here. So I really want people to get this information, to understand how *simple* healing can really be, how *easy* and *pleasant* it can be. But most people won't do it unless they first understand how *dangerous* the present system is. I hope this book has moved you closer to that understanding and increased your willingness to walk away from the lethal dose.

Dr. Jennifer Daniels

RESOURCES

Healing Recipes: http://vitalitycapsules.com/truth-files

Vitality Capsules: http://vitalitycapsules.com/truth-files

Gift for You: Report - *Natural Remedies So Powerful, They May Make Antibiotics Obsolete*. This report details the remedies that made it possible for me to stop prescribing antibiotics altogether in my medical practice. Get it here: http://vitalitycapsules.com/remedies

Discovery Session: http://vitalitycapsules.com/discovery-session-2

Do You Have The Guts To Be Beautiful:
http://vitalitycapsules.com/truth-files

Video: Murder by medicine is no accident:
http://vitalitycapsules.com/death-by-medicine-episode-iii

ENDNOTES

(1) Leape, L. L. 1994. Error in medicine. JAMA 272 (23):1851–7. Null, Gary (2011-10-16). Death by Medicine (p. 177). NBN_Mobi_Kindle. Kindle Edition.

(2) National Patient Safety Foundation (NPSF). Nationwide poll on patient safety: 100 million Americans see medical mistakes directly touching them [press release]. McLean, VA: October 9, 1997. Null, Gary (2011-10-16). Death by Medicine (pp. 177-178). NBN_Mobi_Kindle. Kindle Edition.

(3) COALITION FOR NURSING HOME REFORM. Starfield, B. 2000. Deficiencies in US medical care. JAMA 284 (17):2184–5.

(4) Null, Gary (2011-10-16). Death by Medicine (p. 179). NBN_Mobi_Kindle. Kindle Edition

(5) "Hospital-acquired infections FAQ ." *National Conference of State Legislatures* . National Conference of State Legislatures, n.d. Web. 18 Jun 2013.
<http://www.ncsl.org/issues-research/health/hospital-acquired-infections-faq.aspx/>.

(6) Are We Ready for This Change?: Preventing Pressure Ulcers in Hospitals: A Toolkit for Improving Quality of Care. April 2011. Agency for Healthcare Research and Quality, Rockville, MD.
http://www.ahrq.gov/professionals/systems/long-term-care/resources/pressure-ulcers/pressureulcertoolkit/putool1.html

(7) Brownstein, Catherine A., and John S. Brownstein. "Estimating Excess Mortality in Post-Invasion Iraq." New England Journal of Medicine. Vol. 358 No. 5 (2008): pp. 445-447. Web. 18 Jun. 2013.
<http://www.nejm.org/toc/nejm/358/5/>.

Printed in Great Britain
by Amazon